# The

# Hippopotamus

# Within

## THE HIPPOPOTAMUS DIET

Allen Ekstrom

ISBN: 1497387310
ISBN-13: 978-1497387317

# DEDICATION

This book is dedicated to my Dad, Oscar, to my Uncle George and to all the other Servicemen and Servicewomen who have served to keep America free in the past and present. *Thank you and may God Bless You.*

-Allen Ekstrom

# The Hippopotamus Within

## Table of Contents:

*It's Not Your Fault...*

## ACKNOWLEDGMENT

I would like to acknowledge the owners of **Create**Space for the opportunity they have given me to publish The Hippopotamus Within. Without their help and vision this book would never have been published. To them and their staff I give homage. —Allen Ekstrom

# Chapter One

## Realizations at Hand...

## Circa: 2007

Profile:

Allen Ekstrom: Blonde (used to be, now gray)
Blue Eyes - Swedish
Scottsdale, Arizona, USA
Age: 59
Height: 5-foot 8 inches
Weight: 268 lbs.
Born: 1947... turning 60 in two and a half
months.
Loves: Soda Pop


That's the rap sheet. Do you see anything
wrong with this picture? Two Hundred and
Sixty Eight pounds, that's what's wrong. I had
completely spun out and crashed against the
wall of life going into turn six.

Watching the 2007 NBA Playoffs, the announcer emoted into his microphone: LeBraun James! Six foot eight and 268 pounds! LeBraun is totally unstoppable going to the basket!" Blankly thinking to myself... well, I'm _five_ foot eight and 268! There's only a foot difference between LeBraun and me.

What happened? Why did this happen?

Tell you what... Life happened and I took my eye off the ball. And, waking up one morning 42 years later, realizing my fifties are gone and I am 268 pounds...

I said to myself... It is time to make a change!

So, after taking stock, and putting all the stupid mistakes behind, I'm committing to making the next ten years, 60 to 70, the best 10 years of my life. To do that, the weight needs to go.

Before going on, let's make it clear that I am not a Doctor, or a Psychologist or a Nutritionist... or anything else that takes hard work and study. Some people, after reading this book will be critical of it. But in all probability, those people will be the ones who have something to *sell you*.

I don't have anything to sell you... except my story. And, I'm not telling you or asking you to do what I have done; I am just telling you my story. So with that, let's journey on. It is my hope that you will enjoy the book and know that _you_ can take charge of your life as I did.

# Chapter Two

## It's Not Your Fault

Okay, I'm a fatty. So, whose fault is it anyway, McDonald's? People need to know this so they can make a determination if they should feel bad about themselves or not. We Americans have to assign the blame of every situation to someone, don't we?

Whether it's your spouse laying the blame game or a guilt trip on you, or your mother or father, or son or daughter or your doctor... stop eating!... don't eat that! Put that down, eat an apple!

Why doesn't the good intentioned person say instead, what is it in your life that makes you feel you have to eat like you do? When they say: "don't eat that", it is like saying "stop breathing right now!"

It seems that every good intentioned comment by a friend or loved one pushes you that much farther away from your goal. They are quietly/loudly insulting, and your defenses come up, even if you don't show it outwardly.

Comments like that make you feel bad... or worse yet, may solidify in your own mind that your overweightedness is firmly your fault. When that happens, the next bag of chips comes out and depression seeps in.

The slim, trim, person standing outside of the circle with their arms folded looking down their nose at you says, well, yes, whose fault else could it be? *You* make the decision to put the food in your mouth. *You* are the one making yourself fat... so stop it!

Well, I'm here to tell you that nothing could be farther from the truth.

It's not your fault.

# Chapter Three

## Well Then
## Whose Fault Is It?

Okay, I found myself standing at the edge of the un-harvested fields of time of my sixties. I had this great hope of the best years ahead freshly tucked away in my back pocket.

268 pounds and now what? Okay, deep breath and some thought. Blank. The only thing to think of was... losing weight should be easy!

I was a smart person. I could think. Reduce this to the ridiculous. It's as simple as not putting food in your mouth! Okay, okay, we do have to eat to survive. Okay, modified thought... it's as simple as putting the right foods in your mouth. Better. Could it be that easy?

Well, then a revelation... a celebrity weight loss company spokeswoman was talking on TV one night. She was twirling around squealing with joy saying: "I lost seven pounds in two and a half weeks!" As to which I pondered: how many calories a day can she have?" "1200!" She chirped, answering my question before I could think.

And then it hit. If a mite like her can lose 7 pounds in a couple of weeks, what can a big guy like me lose? So, okay, what kind of foods can be eaten and still keep under 1200 calories per day? My normal regimen called for 3 to 4 thousand calories per day. Hmmm... this was going to be a challenge.

After turning off the TV, I staggered wearily into the bathroom to brush my teeth. While brushing, I happened to glance at myself in the mirror and much to my shock I realized, just for a split second mind you, while hunching over the sink...

*I looked somewhat like a Hippopotamus!*

My senses darted back thinking, WHAT!! This isn't what I look like. I don't look like this. This isn't me. And then another revelation was delivered: I have a Hippopotamus living with me... in me!

## <u>The Hippopotamus Within!</u>

The thought again rushed through my brain. This wasn't me! It was a Hippopotamus! The Hippopotamus made me eat out of control... the Hippopotamus made me the way I am. It's not My Fault!

And, it's Not Your Fault either! I submit to you... that we all have a "Hippopotamus Within", hidden inside us, wanting to control us, to dictate to us, to destroy us! It's the Hippopotamus who really wants to destroy us and make us feel sad about ourselves!

# Chapter Four

## I Fell In Love
## With a Hippopotamus!

It all now made perfect sense, as insane as it sounds. I had fallen in love with a Hippopotamus! The Hippo was a demanding and controlling inner part of me that had taken over. But... he had now been discovered! He had shown himself and I caught him!

I wouldn't do this to myself. This isn't my fault... this is the Hippo's fault! All these years of feeling guilty, beating myself up inside, waging the diet war against myself. Well things have now changed. I know who to blame. I know who to fight... the Hippopotamus within me.

After much reflection, my story with the Hippo had been a sad tale of mayonnaise, ice cream, blue cheese dressing and baked potatoes with dollops of butter and sour cream, double cheese burgers, French fries and that wonderful fried fat found around the edges of my steak.

The Hippo forced me to have relationships with that full strength cola in the red can and greasy potato chips in the big yellow bag. He was sly on that one… he said "I bet you can't eat just one".

I was at the mercy of the Hippo… I ate everything and anything and as much as he told me to. I was, for lack of a better term, the Hippo's "Whipping Boy". The Hippo would force me to have affiliations with Crème Brule, potato salad, and fluffy dinner rolls laden with real creamery butter and jam.

I was so in love, I wanted to look like him and I did a pretty good job of it too. It was much like an abused person who couldn't find the courage all these years to leave the abuser because we both blamed ourselves for our lot in life.

Surely, it wasn't the Hippo's fault that I looked like him... it had to be mine. After all, I did enjoy all of the 3000 - 4000 calorie days I was having.

Why should I look at the calories on the side of the box? If I did, the Hippo might think I didn't trust him. But...I did have my revelation, I cannot deny it. I now knew the truth and I wasn't going to ignore it anymore!

## So, Here Is The Reality... WE ALL HAVE A Hippopotamus Within!

Whether the Hippo is within you for food, drugs, tobacco, alcohol, sex, gambling or shopping, only you can determine. Many fortunate people out there know how to keep their Hippo "In the River" so to speak and don't have problems associated with the aforementioned, so why couldn't I?

Well, I came clean.

I decided I was going to put the Hippo "Back in the River" where he belongs! I was going to put myself back in charge!

# Chapter Five

## What in the World to Do Now?

The American marketing and advertising industries are the finest in the world at what they do. They are big funny money driven machines creating products and services for things you and I never knew we needed. God Bless Them. I admire them. They have turned "the need" for weight loss help into billions of dollars spent each year.

I never knew how complicated it was to lose weight! Let's see... if you take this kind of diet pill (and in the small print it says: *combined with a sensible diet and exercise*) you will lose weight. Huh! How about that... sounds good to me! Who do they think they are kidding?

Or, Infomercials, diet books, exercise programs & fads fueled by the media and movie stars, all written by some authority for our own good. I've often wondered if those slim, trim, authorities ever had to lose a large amount of weight themselves... or did they just urp back at you what they read on the tele-prompter?

My personal favorite was the program that warned that you could have an uncontrolled "accident" (bowel movement) at anytime and to have a change of clothes handy. Whoohoo! Now we're really getting someplace! What is that... an "inter-active" weight loss program?

All I know is that I don't do very well when someone else tells me what to do... like the Hippo. I do much better when it is my idea... I think we all do.

Have you ever felt like you are dying when dieting? Does the word dieting have the word "die" in it? I think it does! So, what in the world should I do now?

Bingo!

# Chapter Six

## Taking Charge Was Liberating

Hahh! With all of this in my mind, the simplest thought hit me. Why don't I just create my own diet program? I figured since I was responsible for putting on the weight, I should be responsible for getting it off. *Unheard of! It can't be done! You are taking a risk! You'll just gain the weight back! You're going to die!*

I shut all of the naysayers out of my mind and you know what? It was very easy. First thing to do was to check with my doctor. After that, I was off and running.

Let's re-visit the TV weight loss celebrity, the one who made me think and gave me inspiration. Okay, the plan was to develop a daily menu with a <u>temporary</u> target of 1200 calories per day. So how is this accomplished?

In a direct confrontation with the Hippopotamus, I raised the courage to start reading the "Nutritional Facts" label on the foods in the supermarket... simple enough. I don't care what the Hippo thinks... I'm sick and tired of pleasing him! I became familiar with how many calories the foods I enjoy had, in proportion to the portions and sought to put them into a menu form.

The internet was a huge help. I went online and typed "foods that burn fat" in the search area. Bingo... up popped a site to list many vegetables, fish and meats.

I could now add the ones I liked to the "menu". Whenever I wanted to know how many calories a certain food had, I just typed in the name of the food and the word "calories" right behind. Several websites appeared, all happy to tell me how many calories were in a certain item.

So okay, I had developed the menu portion of my "Program" and you know what? I liked all of the foods that were on it... because I was in

<u>charge</u> of the menu and not someone else!

I thought to myself, I feel very comfortable about this, maybe I'm on to something here.

# Chapter Seven

## When I Get Hungry... I Will Eat

I started to listen to my inner body. I decided that whenever I get hungry... I will eat ... and whenever I have to go, well, I will go!

So, at the very start of developing my personal program, I made these three rules:

Rule # 1:  When I get hungry... I will always have something to eat - no matter what time of the day or night (watching closely the caloric intake).

Rule #2:  When I have "to go", I will allow myself "to go" as many times as is needed, no matter what time of the day or night.

Rule # 3:  Refer to rule # 2.

Anyway! I am not going to put myself in a self defeating position that would make me feel deprived or frustrated on the way to my goal. After all, the foods I am preparing are <u>my</u> handpicked, low calorie favorites that I enjoy.

Then, the moment of truth happened.

I let go.

My ego handed its power over to my soul. It was instantly liberating to listen to the needs of my body, rather than having the clock say "It's time to eat"! That's right; "the clock says it's time to eat!" was now in limbo. Could I still have lunch with my friends at noon? Of course! I am in control.

I found myself eating smaller portions knowing I could eat whenever I wanted. A confession: Every now and then the target calories for the day were exceeded.

Even though this would happen on occasion, the program overall yielded a system of eating that gave me less stress, guilt and temptation.

# Chapter Eight

## Walk It Off!

One of the late night talk shows was on the tube and an A-List actor was the featured guest. The host and the actor were talking and laughing and the topic came around to weight loss.

The actor leaned back in his chair and then with a confident seriousness in his voice, made back handed waving motions to the audience and said: "If you want to lose weight, just walk it off!"

For some reason, his statement has always stuck. Even before I created my personal weight loss program, I decided that a walk would always start the day.

I first started out by walking "around the block". The "blocks" in my Scottsdale neighborhood were a half a mile long from stop light to stop light. So, a "walk around the block" ended up being two miles.

The walk was a treat as it brought me by many orange and grapefruit trees, & beautiful yards and pools. Its downfall though, was the busy traffic whizzing by my elbow, just a few feet away.

One day, I decided to create a personal, private two mile walking route within the inner neighborhood streets of the original "perimeter block". I got in my car and devised a pleasant, safe, two mile circuit from and to the front door of my lovely little tiled roof flat.

This "private course" became an instant favorite... an "anchor" of mine, if you will. At 6:30 AM there were plenty of cotton tails hopping around. The well manicured yards were an enjoyment to see... and the inner streets were quiet and provided an excellent, protective environment for thought and reflection to organize the day.

Once the personal menu program was started, an extra walk was added in the evening. Since the plan was to lose the weight, the result didn't want me to end up looking like 5 pounds of manure in a 10 pound bag! So, some extra enjoyable exercise was just the ticket.

The second walk would start out around 7:00 PM just as the sun was going behind Camelback Mountain. At the completion of the two miles, the sun would be almost gone and the palm trees would stand out as tall silhouetted sentinels against the fading light of the sky. It was a beautiful and peaceful walk to end the day and it proved to better help induce sleep.

So, an activity had been set up that was truly looked forward to and by doing so, was able to get in 4 miles of exercise per day. By the way, four miles of walking burns off almost an extra 600 calories per day for a guy of my weight!

But wait! There will be of course the weight loss experts who clamor... "We have a program that lets you exercise three times a week for twenty minutes each and get better results than walking!"

But then again, do they really know <u>YOU</u>?  Of course they don't.  They blanket market anyone with a pulse.  An old guy like me might try to do what they say, have a heart attack and drop dead on the spot.

Only you know you... so if that is something that appeals to you, by all means go for it... once again the point is that you are in charge of you.

But keep in mind there is another thing the experts sometimes don't mention and that is stress.  It can almost be guaranteed that exercising three times a week for twenty minutes will not control a full week of stress.

A famed heart specialist said it best and to quote him:  "To get physically tired is the best antidote for nervous tension".

Wa-lah! The truth is powerful stuff! Also, I
had no alcohol, no tobacco, no drugs & no pills to
mess my body up. My plan was and is: plenty
of water, low calorie food of *my* choice and daily
exercise to help me sleep better.

So, again an option for you to consider... Walk
It Off!

# Chapter Nine

## A "Mathematical Certainty"

One way to send the Hippopotamus "Back to the River" is to set up a program that is Fail Safe.

On a Fail Safe program, success would be a by-product of a carefully planned "mathematical certainty", wouldn't it? And by knowing this, it should be much easier to have the courage and determination to follow through knowing success is a certainty.

So, here we go!

The internet has sites that lets you plug in your current weight, height, gender, etc. and tells how many calories it takes to maintain your current weight. It takes 3406 calories, more or less, to maintain my 268 pounds each day with moderate exercise.

Conversely, if you enter a proper "target" weight, it shows the number of daily calories needed to get to and maintain that weight with moderate exercise. I found that it takes 2546 calories every day to get to and maintain my target weight of 180 lbs.

So, assuming moderate activity, if the daily caloric intake is less than 2546 calories, I am on track to achieve my target weight at sometime in the future.

But... wanting to lose the weight a little quicker, I set my program up temporarily for now, taking in no more than 1200 calories on a daily basis. The program was also set up to burn a minimum of 600 calories per day in enjoyable exercise that would reduce stress on a daily basis.

With the goal being a minimum of 1200 calories to a maximum of 2546 calories each day, a "mathematical certainty" of measurable weight loss has been set up.

All that has to be done now is to follow through on a daily basis, be patient, enjoy the results and make the caloric adjustments for maintenance when the target weight is reached.

# Chapter Ten

## The Menu Used

Okay, the personal menus I set up have flexibility and I change them often. Like I said, if I get hungry, I eat! Here is one six portion a day sample menu that I have used. Remember, yours will be different, because <u>you are in control</u> to plug in the foods <u>you like</u> and not me!

Breakfast: Banana 107 calories

              1 cup whole milk 160 cal.

              16-oz. bottled water

Snack:     16-oz. Green Beans 70 cal.

              1 Tb. of light butter 50 cal.

Lunch:     Healthy Choice Entrée 220 Cal.

              16-oz. bottled water

Snack:      5 stalks steamed broccoli 50 cal.

            1 Tb. of light butter 50 cal.

            16-oz. bottled water

Supper:     2 oz. Spaghetti 200 cal.

            1/2 cup Spaghetti sauce 60 cal.

            1 Roma Tomato 35 Cal.

            1/3 cucumber 20 cal.

            16 -oz. Lite Cranberry juice 80 cal.

Snack:      6 sugar free Popsicle single pops @

            15 cal. Ea. 90 calories

            16-oz. bottled water

Total Calories: 1192

The sugar free Popsicle pops were my secret
"ally". I could have just about as many of them
as I wanted and it didn't hurt me calorie wise
during the day. When I thought of food, I'd
"pop" one in my mouth... 15 calories, big deal!

# Chapter Eleven

## Plan for Disaster

Okay, the program was coming together... a daily 1200 to 2546 calorie menu of foods (supplemented with a name brand vitamin pill) that are handpicked favorites... and the authority to eat whenever hungry.

Also, a great non demanding walking course used twice daily for private time, a calorie burner and stress reducer.

And, "The Hippopotamus Within" had been identified and was being dealt with on a daily basis. It was not me to blame for the overweight mess I was in... it was the Hippopotamus and I was now calling the shots!

But as good as the program was going, falling off the wagon and pigging out uncontrollably at some point in time was a certain possibility that had to be contended with. A safety valve had to be set up... A "Plan for Disaster" had to be implemented!

So, a forced "pig out" activity was created. As a "reward" for staying on the program during the week, I "allow" myself to take my dear wife out to dinner every Friday.

Whether to the Buffet, to Chinese or Seafood, we go out and eat. I am allowed to eat what I want and as much as I want. This activity kills two birds with one stone. I'm on my program and I get to spend time with my wife.

If I pig out... so what? As long as it is for just one meal a week, it is a great reward for waging the war against the Hippo the other six and two-thirds days.

Surprisingly, I find I am not pigging out as much as I had given myself the authority to do. This "reward" unknowingly provides a "mental out"... a much needed trusted step in responsible eating on my own.

It is kind of like "parole".  The prisoner that I have been for the Hippopotamus was now starting to get a glimpse of the "outside world"... and it looked good.

# Chapter Twelve

## The Hippopotamus Recap

Well, after two short months, a total of 30 pounds has been lost and it has been pleasant! Weight wise, thirty pounds is seven and a half 4 pound bags of sugar. Try holding those in your arms all at once! That's a lot of weight! Suits that had hung in the closet for years now fit. Breathing is easier and more energy is at hand.

The journey has just begun though, and it will continue. I have set up my vehicle. My program has become a part of my life, it is enjoyable and all of the benefits that will yet unfold as the journey progresses over the years are yet to come!

UPDATE! Fast Forward –Now, in December 2013, I'm at 198 lbs. 70 lbs. less than 2007. I haven't hit my target of 180 lbs, yet... but I did take off 40 more lbs!  And 70 total lbs. are still off!  If I can do this, you can do this!

Are you going to make a program for yourself?  If you do, what will be in your program if you had one?  What are some benefits that may come into your life if you can achieve your target weight?  Some may be new or strengthened love; respect, surprise, shock, envy, new job, a promotion, or a whole new world!

## Okay... Let's Do a Re-cap of

## How I've "Kept the Hippopotamus in the River"!

I made a profile of myself.  I didn't feel guilty about the mistakes of the past, I just released them!  I gave myself more credit than I did before.  I set a target weight goal.

I grabbed my second chance at life.  I didn't blame myself anymore... I blamed the Hippopotamus!  I decided what I was going to do and then just did it. I set up a program that is comfortable and measurable. I tried new menus... and sought out new favorite foods.

I always eat when I'm hungry and I go when I have to! I "Walked It Off!" I set up a routine I look forward to. I set up a personal "Mathematical Certainty," it's easy! I made a "Plan for "Disaster" by rewarding myself! I don't do what the Hippopotamus tells me anymore!

*I Put the Hippo "Back In the River"!*

# Chapter Thirteen

## Well, That About Does It!

Please keep in mind that I have told you my story... what I am doing. I'm not telling *you* what to do or how to do it because I don't know you.

Here's what I can tell you though. If you want to lose weight, first get a check up with your doctor and seek his or her advice before you start. My doctor suggested a vitamin pill supplement every day when I started.

No one knows you better than you and sometimes blanket diet plans, pills or exercise machines cannot serve the needs of everyone as we are all different and have different needs.

Stop and listen to your body... stop and have some quiet time for you. Give yourself more credit than you are giving yourself. Take a hand in your destiny. We are all on a journey... make it fun with a new healthy you.

I will close with a quote from a poster I saw at an airport in Chicago.

It said...

*"There Are Those Who Jump Puddles...*

*Then There Are Those Who Jump Oceans...*

*It's Time to Fly"!*
--------------------------

# Let's Fly!

*Thank You and May God Bless You*

*On Your Journey in Life!*

*-Allen Ekstrom*

# Chapter Fourteen

## Some Foods That Burn Fat

Abalone - Bass - Catfish - Clams - Chives - Onions - Leeks - Scallions - Shallots - Pumpkin - Squash - Garlic - Soybeans - Bananas - Dairy Products - Cod Crab - Crayfish - Buffalo Fish - Flounder - Frog Legs Lobster - Mussels - Grapefruit - Kumquats - Lemons Limes - Mangoes - Nectarines - Oranges - Papaya - Pears Peaches - Pineapple - Pomegranates - Prunes - Quince Tangerines - Green Beans - Green Peppers - Kohlrabi Mushrooms - Okra - Peas - Red Peppers - Rhubarb - Salsify - Oysters - Sea Bass - Shrimp - Steaks - String Beans - Tomatoes - Carrots - Parsnips - Radishes Rutabagas - Turnips - Cantaloupe - Honeydews Muskmelon - Watermelon - Cabbage - Chinese Cabbage

Dandelion Greens - Belgian Endive - Sorrel -
Spinach Watercress - Blackberries - Blueberries
- Cranberries Currants - Strawberries -
Huckleberries - Loganberries Raspberries -
Grapes - Apples - Apricots – Cherries - Plums -
Terrapin - Trout - Tuna - Corn - Cucumbers
and... Eggplant!

# Chapter Fifteen

## Walking Chart

### Calories Burned Per Mile

| Speed/Pounds | 100 lb | 120 lb | 140 lb | 160 lb | 180 lb | 200 lb | 220 lb | 250 lb | 275 lb | 300 lb |
|---|---|---|---|---|---|---|---|---|---|---|
| 2.0mph | 57 | 68 | 80 | 91 | 102 | 114 | 125 | 142 | 156 | 170 |
| 2.5mph | 55 | 65 | 76 | 87 | 98 | 109 | 120 | 136 | 150 | 164 |
| 3.0mph | 53 | 64 | 74 | 85 | 95 | 106 | 117 | 133 | 146 | 159 |
| 3.5mph | 52 | 62 | 73 | 83 | 94 | 104 | 114 | 130 | 143 | 156 |
| 4.0mph | 57 | 68 | 80 | 91 | 102 | 114 | 125 | 142 | 156 | 170 |
| 4.5mph | 64 | 76 | 89 | 10 | 11 | 12 | 14 | 159 | 175 | 191 |

| | | | 2 | 5 | 7 | 0 | | | |
|---|---|---|---|---|---|---|---|---|---|
| 5.0mph | 73 | 87 | 102 | 116 | 131 | 145 | 160 | 182 | 200 | 218 |

The chart of calories burned per mile is based on MET research - metabolic equivalents of various activities.

References: AINSWORTH BE, Haskell WL, Whitt MC, Irwin ML, Swartz AM, Strath SJ, O'Brien WL, Bassett DR Jr, Schmitz KH, Emplaincourt PO, Jacobs DR Jr, Leon AS. "Compendium of Physical Activities: An update of activity codes and MET intensities." Med Sci Sports Exerc 2000; 32 (Suppl):S498-S516.

www.ingramcontent.com/pod-product-compliance
Lightning Source LLC
Chambersburg PA
CBHW070338290526
45791CB00003B/1382